Hysterectomy Vaginal Repair

FOURTH EDITION

Sally Haslett
RGN, RM, RHV, FPCert

and

Molly Jennings
MCSP, SRP

BEACONSFIELD PUBLISHERS LTD
Beaconsfield, Bucks, UK

First published 1984
Fourth edition 1998
© Sally Haslett and Molly Jennings 1984, 1988, 1992, 1998

British Library Cataloguing in Publication Data

Haslett, Sally
    Hysterectomy and vaginal repair – 4th ed.
    1. Hysterectomy – Popular works   2. Vagina –Surgery – Popular works
    I. Title   II. Jennings, Molly
    618.1'453

    ISBN 0–906584–46–9

Medical artwork: Barbara Hyams
Photography: Mike Messer
Photographic models: Elizabeth Pearson MCSP and Judy Difiore

Phototypeset by Gem Graphics, Trenance, Mawgan Porth, Cornwall
in 10¾ on 12 point Times.
Printed in Great Britain at The Bath Press, Bath.

From the Foreword to the First Edition

Not all doctors are good communicators and many patients in clinics are poor listeners. This is particularly true when they are nervous or worried and faced with the prospect of surgery. At least, many fail to ask all of the questions that may concern them later. When the operation appears to carry the threat to sexual function, the worries can be particularly hard to put into words.

Some years ago, in the gynaecological department of St Thomas' Hospital, we attempted to meet this problem by asking two women staff members, who themselves had undergone major gynaecological surgery, to try to explore and relieve the anxieties of women about to have a hysterectomy, or repair surgery for prolapse. The experience was an unqualified success and has contributed greatly to post-operative wellbeing – particularly the long-term mental and physical wellbeing that hospital doctors often ignore.

From this experience Sally Haslett and Molly Jennings have produced this booklet and I recommend that every woman who faces such surgery should now read it. I have no doubt that it will lessen her anxieties and speed her recovery.

R. W. Taylor MD, FRCOG
Professor Emeritus, Department of Obstetrics and Gynaecology
St Thomas' Hospital, London

Contents

INTRODUCTION

When women are advised to have a hysterectomy and/or vaginal repair they are often reluctant to ask questions about their diagnosis, the surgery to be performed and the convalescent period. This may be due to a lack of understanding of the anatomy of their reproductive organs, but may also be due to embarrassment over the intimate and private nature of their problem. They may simply not know what questions to ask, or feel that what they would like to ask is too basic. It is often easier to obtain this information by having a book to read.

This booklet provides information about these operations and will be useful for reference, both before and after the surgery.

UNDERSTANDING YOUR BODY

First of all, it is important that you should fully understand your anatomy and the terminology used in relation to specific organs (Figures 1, 2, 3 and 4, overleaf). The reproductive organs are contained within the pelvic girdle – that is, the ring of bones formed by the two large hip bones, the base of the spine (sacrum) and tail bone (coccyx) at the back and the pubic bone at the front, under the pubic hair. The top rim of the pelvic girdle can be felt about 5 cm (2 inches) below the waist on either side. The reproductive organs are:

The Ovaries
The ovaries are situated deep in the pelvis on either side of the womb and contain a large number of eggs. In women of childbearing age, one egg is usually released each month and enters the fallopian tube, where it may become fertilised and pass to the womb.

The Fallopian Tubes (Salpinges)
These open into the womb, one on either side. They have a thick lining, with the ability to help the egg travel along them and enter the womb.

The Womb (Uterus)
The womb is about the size and shape of a small pear (5–8 cm or 2–3 inches long), wide at the top and narrower below, and lies just behind the pubic bone. It is made up of layers of muscle and is lined with special tissue called endometrium, which has a large blood supply. The ligaments,

1

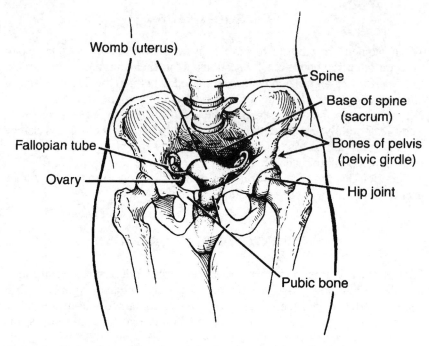

Figure 1   *Front view of female pelvis showing position of womb (uterus) in the body.*

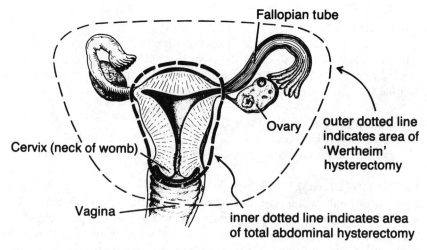

Figure 2   *Front view of womb (uterus).*

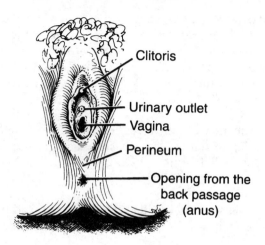

Figure 3   *Female genital area.*

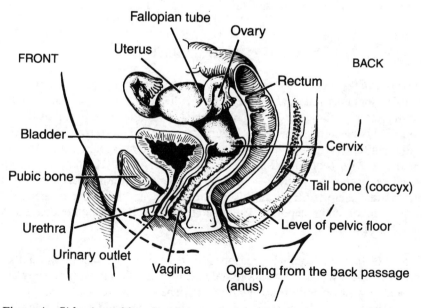

Figure 4   *Side view of female pelvic area, showing pelvic organs and pelvic floor muscles.*

3

acting like ropes, hold the womb in position within the pelvis. The function of the womb is to expand to hold a developing baby. Each month, during a woman's reproductive life, the lining of the womb prepares to receive a fertilised egg for it to implant and grow. If this does not happen, the lining is shed by the normal blood loss of the monthly period (menstruation).

The Cervix

The narrow entrance at the 'neck' or base of the womb is called the cervix. This is a ring of muscle that can relax and open to allow a baby to pass through during childbirth.

The Vagina

The vagina is sometimes called the birth canal and the cervix dips down into it. The vaginal walls are muscular and very elastic, so stretch easily.

The External Genital Area (Vulva)

The part between the legs into which the vagina opens is called the genital area or vulva. The lips on either side surround the openings from the urethra/urinary canal at the front and from the vagina just behind. The perineum separates the vulva from the anus (Figure 3).

HYSTERECTOMY

The word 'hysterectomy' means having the womb (uterus) removed. It usually includes removal of the neck of the womb (cervix), i.e. a 'total hysterectomy'; if the cervix is not removed, it is called a sub-total hysterectomy. Hysterectomy may also involve removal of either or both of the fallopian tubes (right or left or bilateral salpingectomy) and either or both of the ovaries (oophorectomy) (Figures 1, 2, and 4). Having the womb removed brings the obvious advantage of no more monthly periods. It also means that there is no possibility of pregnancy, and therefore no need for any form of contraception. The operation may be recommended for a number of reasons:

Fibroids (a very common reason for hysterectomy). These are bulky growths of muscle and fibrous tissue that form inside the womb. They are almost always benign (not malignant). They increase the area of the lining of the womb, often causing heavy bleeding and painful periods, although occasionally there may be no symptoms. In certain circumstances fibroids can be removed, leaving the womb intact. The operation is called 'myomectomy'. (The practical advice on recovery and after-care given in this booklet also applies following myomectomy.)

Dysfunctional Bleeding or Menorrhagia. Here a woman experiences heavy and prolonged bleeding. It may be irregular, often with clots of blood, and can cause her to be anaemic and complain of extreme tiredness. Hysterectomy is usually only considered after other treatments have been unsuccessful.

Endometriosis (chocolate cysts) – a spread of the tissue that lines the womb to areas other than the lining of the womb, e.g. the ovaries and fallopian tubes. This tissue attempts to shed blood each month and painful cysts may form. It often gives rise to severe pain associated with the monthly period, and a heavy blood loss.

Pelvic Inflammatory Disease (PID). This is an infection of the fallopian tubes and other pelvic organs, often recurring, and causing low abdominal pain.

Prolapse (see pages 8–9).

Tumours. In some cases surgery is performed to remove tumours, the vast majority of which are 'benign' or harmless. Cancer is very rarely the reason for hysterectomy. However, it may occur in the cervix, the lining of the womb, or in one or both ovaries. A woman may complain of some unusual bleeding or discharge, increased tummy size, pain, or may in fact have no symptoms. When cancer is diagnosed an extended or 'Wertheim's' hysterectomy will normally be performed. This usually involves removal of the ovaries and fallopian tubes, adjacent glands and the upper third of the vagina, as well as the womb (Figures 2, 3 and 4). Any tissue removed is always sent to the laboratory for analysis. (Occasionally only a small sample of a suspect area is taken for analysis, and this is called a 'biopsy'.)

Should any form of cancer be discovered, surgery and probably chemotherapy and/or radiotherapy may be recommended. For specific advice or more detailed information, refer to the sources given in 'Additional Reading' (page 35).

When a Hysterectomy is Recommended

The doctor should explain fully his or her decision for this advice and women should be encouraged to ask questions at this stage – even requesting another opinion if necessary. *It is important to feel fully informed and understand exactly what the operation means.* You may find it helpful to write down your questions beforehand and possibly take a friend with you for support.

Frequently, symptoms such as heavy bleeding or pain will have been experienced, and a hysterectomy offers a welcome cure and the opportunity of improved health, without impairment of a woman's sexuality.

A hysterectomy is no reason (or excuse!) for gaining or losing weight, neither is it a cause of depression or any other character change or loss of femininity, although this is a fear of many women.

If the operation is performed before the menopause (change of life) and the ovaries left intact, hormones will continue to be produced. Menstrual cycle symptoms, if previously experienced, may therefore continue (such as breast tenderness, feeling 'bloated', irritability or depression at certain times of the month). These symptoms, however, are usually less intense than before and will end with the natural menopause (see pages 31–2).

If the ovaries are *both* removed, symptoms of the menopause may follow unless the hormones are replaced artificially, i.e. by hormone replacement therapy (HRT) (see pages 32–3).

Hysterectomy may be performed either through an abdominal incision ('total or sub-total abdominal hysterectomy') or vaginally ('vaginal hysterectomy'). It is also possible that laparoscopic surgery may be recommended (see below).

An *abdominal* incision is usually a horizontal 'bikini-line' along the top of the pubic hair line, and this leaves little or no perceptible scar. For some patients, particularly those with large fibroids or who are overweight, the incision may be made vertically on the lower abdomen. Abdominal incisions are closed either with stitches or clips. (For removal, see 'Wound Care', page 13.)

It may be possible to remove the womb *vaginally*. This is frequently advised where there is a 'prolapsed' womb and a vaginal repair is also needed. With vaginal surgery (Figures 3 and 4) there is no visible incision, and the surgery is repaired with stitches that dissolve. A vaginal hysterectomy may not be possible where the womb is enlarged, or if the surgeon wishes to look closely at other pelvic or abdominal organs while operating.

Hysterectomy

Laparoscopically-Assisted Surgery. 'Keyhole' or laparoscopically-assisted surgery may be advised where appropriate. This simply means that the surgeon is helped by the use of a laparoscope – a very fine tube with a light and a type of small magnifying glass at the tip. An anaesthetic is given and the laparoscope is slipped in through a small cut on your abdomen.

When this procedure is carried out, three or four small cuts may be made. Harmless gas is pumped in to raise your abdominal wall and make it easier for the doctor to see your pelvic organs – rather like working in a bell-tent! It is most commonly used to assist a vaginal hysterectomy.

You may feel a little distended and bruised for a day or two afterwards, mainly due to pressure from the gas on your internal organs. This will eventually be absorbed and disappear. Pain in the right shoulder, due to gas trapped under the rib cage, may also be a problem; normally a few deep breaths will help to relieve it, but if it persists, seek medical advice.

The small cuts on your abdomen will usually be closed with one or two stitches. These may dissolve or need to be removed after five days, probably at your own doctor's surgery. After this type of hysterectomy, the recovery period is usually much shorter than after conventional surgery. It is wise to ask your doctor's advice in each individual case.

An abdominal hysterectomy can involve fairly extensive internal surgery. This means that although externally the scar will heal quickly – usually within a week – the internal healing process takes considerably longer. The time for recovery depends very much on the type and extent of the surgery, your general health, state of mind, and a careful life style during your convalescence.

Some women experience difficulty in coming to terms with having a hysterectomy. Others find they are affected emotionally after the operation. The understanding support of family and friends can be invaluable at this time, but 'counselling', or time for discussion with a sympathetic and informed health professional, can do much to dispel myths and alleviate anxiety. It is important that both the woman concerned and her family are able to obtain *accurate* information about this operation in advance. A list of useful addresses and additional reading material which may be helpful is given on pages 34–5.

VAGINAL REPAIR FOR PROLAPSE AND URINARY INCONTINENCE

A 'vaginal repair' is the operation performed to correct a 'prolapse'. A prolapse occurs when the supporting sling (or ligaments) which holds the womb and other pelvic organs in position is no longer strong enough to do this effectively. The womb may descend or 'drop down' in varying positions, pressing on other pelvic organs such as the bladder or bowel, and resulting in different types of prolapse (see Figures 5, 6 and 7). The sling (or ligaments), the walls of the vagina, and the pelvic floor muscles (Figure 4) may become weakened for various reasons, the most common being pregnancy and childbirth.

Other causes may be a chronic cough (as with smokers or people with bronchitis), straining when constipated, continuous heavy lifting, or following the menopause when the decrease in production of female hormones affects the elasticity of the tissues.

A prolapse may be described as 'something coming down' in the vagina. It may cause backache and difficulty in controlling the bladder and sometimes the bowel, or discomfort during intercourse.

The surgery to repair a prolapse is often combined with a hysterectomy, in which case the womb is usually removed vaginally and the vaginal walls are strengthened and repaired at the same time, using stitches which dissolve.

If the womb is *not* removed, the sling (or ligaments) will be shortened to lift the womb back into place. This will allow the bladder and bowel to return to their correct position. The supporting muscles (pelvic floor muscles) may also need repair due to the stretching.

Occasionally these muscles and the vaginal walls need repairing at some time *after* a woman has had a hysterectomy – especially if she has not continued with her pelvic floor exercises (as described on pages 19–20). These exercises will not cure a prolapse but are of great value *before* and *after* surgery, by strengthening the supporting pelvic floor muscles.

A repair for prolapse would not usually be advised until a woman has decided that she does not want any more children. However, 'repair' surgery can be performed without removing the womb. In this case periods, and therefore the possibility of pregnancy, will continue in women who have not yet reached the menopause, and contraception will still be necessary if they are sexually active. If pregnancy does occur, the baby will need to be delivered by caesarean section.

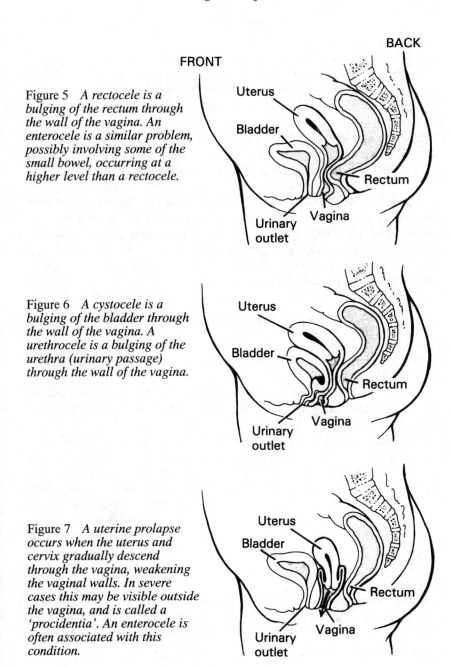

FRONT

BACK

Figure 5   *A rectocele is a bulging of the rectum through the wall of the vagina. An enterocele is a similar problem, possibly involving some of the small bowel, occurring at a higher level than a rectocele.*

Uterus

Bladder

Rectum

Vagina

Urinary outlet

Figure 6   *A cystocele is a bulging of the bladder through the wall of the vagina. A urethrocele is a bulging of the urethra (urinary passage) through the wall of the vagina.*

Uterus

Bladder

Rectum

Vagina

Urinary outlet

Figure 7   *A uterine prolapse occurs when the uterus and cervix gradually descend through the vagina, weakening the vaginal walls. In severe cases this may be visible outside the vagina, and is called a 'procidentia'. An enterocele is often associated with this condition.*

Uterus

Bladder

Rectum

Vagina

Urinary outlet

9

COLPOSUSPENSION

Colposuspension is another operation that may be chosen for problems with control of urine. It involves lifting and holding the neck of the bladder into a new and corrected position. It is usually performed through a bikini-line abdominal incision as for hysterectomy.

Collagen injections are placed at the bladder neck to correct mild incontinence and may be an alternative to colposuspension. This can be done as an outpatient in a day-care unit, usually under local anaesthetic.

The advice in this booklet with regard to recovery following operation applies *equally to hysterectomy, repair surgery and colposuspension.*
A woman undergoing repair surgery will usually have experienced some degree of discomfort and difficulty in controlling her bladder and bowel functions, and possibly also backache. Following surgery, women can look forward to a greatly improved quality of life.

PREPARE FOR YOUR OPERATION

Exercises and Advice
Practise getting in and out of bed correctly, as described and illustrated on pages 16–17.
You may find it helpful to practise deep breathing (page 14) and the pelvic floor exercise (pages 19–20). Follow the advice for housework, ironing and using the vacuum cleaner (page 26).
In general, try not to get too tired before admission. It will also be a good idea to plan ahead for your return home. Try to arrange some help with everyday tasks such as shopping for food and keeping your home in order during your convalescent time. Remember yourself too – plan ahead for any pastimes you enjoy during your convalescent period. Also, check with the hospital when visitors will be welcome. You will be discharged when medical care is no longer necessary, i.e. 3 to 6 days after your surgery, so try to arrange some help at home for your convalescence.

Smoking
If you do smoke, try not to smoke for *at least* three days before and after your operation. Prior to an anaesthetic it is particularly important to have your lungs free from cigarette smoke. Remember that most hospitals now have a no-smoking policy.

ADMISSION TO HOSPITAL

You may be admitted on the day before your operation or on the actual day, or be asked to attend for a pre-admission assessment. On admission, do not hesitate to raise any last-minute worries or anxieties you may have. Remember to tell the hospital staff if you have taken any medicines or drugs recently or have any allergies, whether you have any caps or crowns in your teeth, and whether you require a special diet (for example, diabetic or low fat, etc.).

To prepare you for your operation you will be given nothing to eat or drink for several hours beforehand. The nursing staff will want to ensure that your bowels are empty and may wish to clip or shave hair from your pubic area. You might prefer to ask in advance exactly what will be required and do this for yourself at home. Blood and urine samples will be taken and tested.

It is usual to have a bath or shower before going to the operating theatre and you will also be asked to remove contact lenses, false teeth, make-up, nail varnish and jewellery. You may also be seen by a doctor and you will probably be given a 'pre-med' injection to help you relax.

It is *not* wise to bring valuables, jewellery or a large amount of money into hospital. Just have some small change for the telephone and newspapers. Remember that your concentration is likely to be low after an anaesthetic, so think about bringing something easy to read.

GENERAL CARE AFTER YOUR OPERATION

Pain Relief
The degree of pain or discomfort experienced by patients following surgery varies a great deal. Bruising and soreness around the area of the wound may extend to include the whole genital area following surgery, but should ease after a few days. Injections may be offered initially to relieve pain, then pain-killing tablets are usually sufficient to reduce the discomfort. Pain relief may also be obtained by using rectal suppositories.

Patient-Controlled Analgesia (PCA)
This may be offered for certain operations. A small device is attached to your arm or hand, which enables you to obtain pain relief when you need it. You will be given full information from the hospital if it is appropriate for you.

Depression, or 'Post-Op Blues'

It is not uncommon to feel emotional or weepy immediately following surgery. Many women experience these feelings, but usually only for a day or two. Don't be surprised if these feelings come back when you get home, having left the reassurance of a hospital setting. They are a normal reaction and should pass quickly.

Food and Drink (including 'drips')

For a few hours or longer following your operation it may be necessary to give fluid intravenously (through a drip into a vein – usually in the arm), although you should soon be eating and drinking normally. You may be advised to drink plenty of fluids following your operation, once this is permitted. Until then, do ask for a mouthwash if you need it.

You may experience feelings of nausea. Not everyone has this problem but if you do, tell the medical or nursing staff, who can help to relieve it.

Bladder Care

Everyone differs as to when their normal bladder function is restored. Passing urine usually presents no problem, although flow can sometimes be slow at first due to bruising. You should be allowed to walk to the toilet or use a commode soon after the operation, but a tube or catheter may be left in the bladder to drain the urine in order to rest the repaired tissues. This causes very little discomfort and is removed as soon as possible. You are likely to be encouraged to drink plenty of fluids following the operation, as this will help to prevent any urinary infections.

Bowels and Wind

It is quite normal not to have a bowel motion for the first three or four days after the operation, as the nurses will have ensured that your bowels are empty beforehand. The nurse will give you a laxative if necessary, because straining should be avoided. You may find that it helps to support the area between your legs just in front of your back passage with a pad when passing a bowel motion or wind. Wind may be a real problem – the nursing staff can advise on how to relieve the discomfort, possibly by a peppermint-type 'cocktail'. It may be helped by the pelvic tilting or the knee-rolling exercise described on pages 20–1, or by walking, if allowed.

Some women experience pain in the right shoulder. This is a 'referred' pain caused by the accumulation of wind in the tummy (abdomen). A few slow deep breaths in and out may help to relieve it. *Always tell the nursing staff if you have shoulder pain.*

Wound Care

Thin drainage tubes may be left in place following surgery to remove any excess fluid which may collect beneath the wound. The drained fluid (which is likely to be bloodstained) runs into a small bottle. The tubes are removed when all drainage has ceased – usually 24 to 48 hours after your operation.

Abdominal stitches and clips are normally removed between the fourth and sixth day after the operation. This should not be a painful procedure. Some abdominal stitches, particularly those used to close a small wound, are 'soluble' and will dissolve completely when the area is healed. Numbness or a loss of sensation to touch may be experienced afterwards in the area around the scar tissue. The stitches used inside the vagina are also soluble.

The healing appears rapid on the outside, but it must be remembered that all the many layers of muscle and tissue have to heal internally and this takes much longer.

Circulation, and Prevention of Thrombosis

You may be asked to wear support stockings for a while to help prevent the risk of thrombosis (blood clots in your blood vessels). Nowadays anticoagulant injections are given until you are up and moving freely, to prevent thrombosis. They are not particularly painful but do produce small bruises. This is nothing to worry about.

To improve the circulation in your legs, bend your feet up and down at the ankle, firmly and quickly several times each hour (Figure 8). Also gently bend and stretch your legs one at a time. Do these exercises in bed and also when you are sitting in a chair. When sitting, avoid pressure on the back of your knees by using a footstool if necessary. Do not sit with your legs crossed, as it is bad for the circulation.

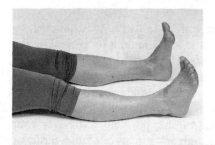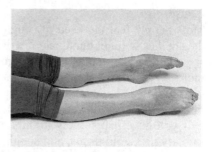

Figure 8   *To improve circulation: legs straight, bend and stretch ankles.*

13

Also, tighten the strong muscles on the front of the thigh by pressing the knee back against the bed whilst pointing your toes towards the ceiling; hold for a few seconds and let go like a pumping movement.

Do this as often as possible, either sitting in a chair or standing. This will not only improve the circulation, but will help to prevent your legs feeling 'wobbly'/weak in the early days after your operation.

Deep Breathing

This helps to reduce the effect of the anaesthetic. Start as soon as you wake up. Sit up in bed, supported by pillows, knees bent up, feet flat on the bed (Figure 9). Take a deep breath in, fill your lungs with air, and sigh the breath out.

Do this three or four times every hour. Remember also to do this breathing exercise when you are sitting out of bed in a chair.

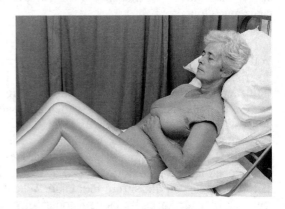

Figure 9
Deep breathing in bed.

Coughing

Most people feel the need to cough after an anaesthetic. It is quite safe – the stitches will not burst, and it will hurt less if you do it properly. Use the same sitting position as for deep breathing. If you have had an abdominal incision, put your hands or forearms over the wound, or cuddle a pillow to your tummy (Figure 10); take a deep breath in and then cough, spitting any mucus out. Repeat as you feel it necessary.

If you have had surgery through your vagina, put your hand over your sanitary pad, hold firmly, and cough, spitting any mucus out into a tissue or container. Do this three or four times or until your chest feels clear.

14

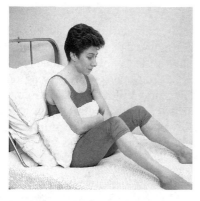
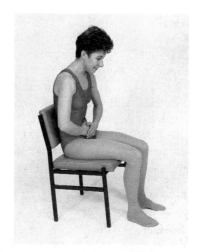

Figure 10   *Coughing, showing position
of hands, with or without a pillow: (a) in
bed; (b) sitting in a chair.*

Back Care in Bed

When sitting up in bed, make sure you have a pillow in the middle of your
lower back to maintain the normal hollow at waist level (Figure 11).

Lie flat at night, with pillows under your head, but no back rest. Lie
either on your back or side, whichever is the most comfortable. If you lie
on your side, try cuddling a pillow to support your tummy, and another in
the small of your back.

Figure 11
Back care in bed.

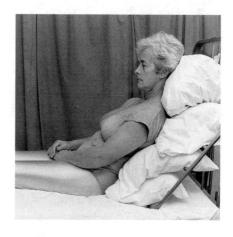

15

Rest

Rest is essential as part of the healing process, both during the day as well as at night. Try to have at least one hour during the day. As just mentioned above, lie with pillows under your head, but no back rest, either on your back or side, whichever is more comfortable. You may find that lying on your side with your knees bent up, or leaning on a pillow cuddled to your tummy, will help to support your stitches. After vaginal surgery you may also find that lying face down with a pillow at waist level is comfortable and rests your back. Keep visitors to a minimum during the first few days, as they can be quite exhausting.

Turning over in Bed

Bend your knees up, keeping them pressed together. Roll over with shoulders and knees in line, so that you do not twist. Think of your body as a log of wood – turning over in this way protects the wound and is less painful.

Getting out of Bed

Bend your knees up, roll onto your side keeping your knees together, push yourself up to a sitting position with your hands, allowing your legs to swing down to the floor (Figure 12). (Reverse this process to get back into bed.)

Gradually, stand up straight, wait for a few seconds to get used to your upright position, and then begin to walk. 'Stand tall' and 'walk tall' – if you have abdominal stitches this will not interfere with their healing.

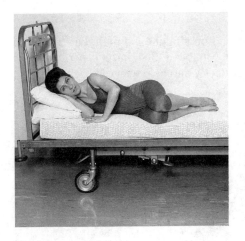
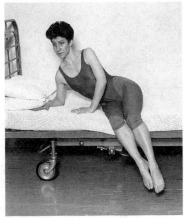

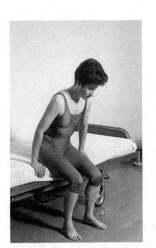
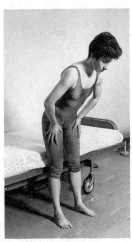
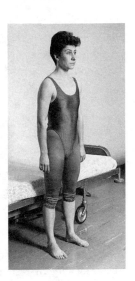

Figure 12   *Getting out of bed: (a) Roll to side, knees together, note position of hands (see 'Turning over in Bed'); (b) Swing legs down, keeping knees bent, and push up with hands to sitting position; (c) Sit on side of bed, feet apart and flat on floor; (d) Lean forward, straighten knees, and stand up; (e) Stand up straight before beginning to walk.*

Posture
Remember – 'walk tall'. Always stand up straight and pull your tummy in (Figure 13). You may find this uncomfortable at first, but it is perfectly safe and will allow the wound to heal correctly and help to avoid backache.

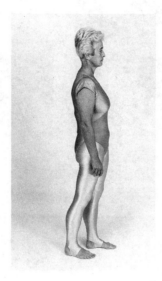

Figure 13
'Walk tall'.

Hygiene
A daily bath or shower will be encouraged following the operation. If you have abdominal stitches you must dry this area well until they dissolve or are removed.

Vaginal Bleeding or Discharge
A slight vaginal discharge is normal for up to six weeks following hysterectomy or repair. It is possible for the discharge to contain threads from dissolving internal vaginal stitches. If the discharge becomes bright red, heavy or with clots, please rest and *seek medical advice at once*. Use sanitary pads. **Do not** use tampons, because of the possibility of introducing infection into the vagina. Only pads should be used, and these should be changed regularly.

EXERCISES FROM THE FIRST DAY AFTER YOUR OPERATION

The Pelvic Floor

The pelvic floor muscles form a sling which passes from the tail bone (coccyx) at the back to the pubic bone at the front of the pelvic girdle (Figures 1 and 4). This sling, or hammock, is in two halves which fan out on either side. It joins at the middle with a gap at the front to allow the back passage (anus), outlet from the womb (vagina) and urinary passage (urethra) to pass through. It is important to keep this sling of muscles like a piece of new elastic. This will enable them to support the abdominal organs efficiently, and by their reflex action to control leaks of urine on sudden movement – for example, on coughing, laughing, running for a bus or at an exercise class.

Pelvic Floor Exercise

Check first with your doctor or physiotherapist how soon you may begin this exercise after colposuspension or vaginal repair.

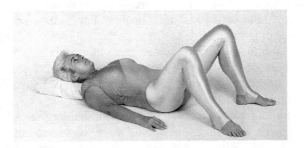

Figure 14   *Pelvic floor exercise in lying position.*

The pelvic floor exercise is a very important one and should be started as soon as possible. It may be done in any position – for example, lying with knees bent up (Figure 14), sitting in a chair, or in a standing position once you are allowed to get up.

The aim of the exercise is to contract or tighten the pelvic floor muscles. This is a feeling rather like stopping the passing of wind at the same time as stopping a loss of urine. It is a lifting and squeezing movement, and should not involve the tummy or buttock muscles.

Keeping your legs slightly apart, and remembering to breathe normally, draw up and close your back passage. At the same time draw up and close your vagina and urinary passage. Hold this contraction for as many seconds as you can, and then let go. Rest briefly between contractions. Gradually try – over days or even weeks – to increase the length of the contraction or 'hold' up to 8–10 seconds, if possible. Repeat as many times as you can – the pelvic floor muscles tire easily, so stop when you find your ability to hold is becoming weaker. Rest and try again later.

Aim to do your pelvic floor exercise at frequent intervals during the day. To test that you are doing it correctly, try occasionally to stop the flow of urine in mid-stream – but *never* do this more than once or twice a week.

When you are confident you are doing the exercise correctly, it is important to add up to ten fast one-second contractions at least once each day, in order to involve all the types of muscle fibres which make up the pelvic floor. Make these short contractions as strong as possible.

The Abdominal Muscles

The abdominal (tummy) muscles form an elastic corset. They help to hold the abdominal organs in their correct place and so aid digestion. These muscles also act as a 'splint' for the back – this helps to protect your spine, and will help you to maintain a good posture. Fat is attracted to the tissues between the abdominal muscle layers and so attention to diet is important.

All these gentle exercises are designed to strengthen the abdominal muscles and are of particular value following abdominal surgery. Do not worry if you find them difficult at first – they will become easier with each day.

First, try pulling your tummy muscles in and holding for a few seconds, and let go slowly. Remember not to hold your breath and not to raise your shoulders. Do this as often as you can – 3 or 4 times at first, then rest. Do it in bed, sitting in a chair, standing or walking. It is a gentle exercise, but safe and easy to do and will help regain the strength and elasticity of very important muscles.

Pelvic Tilting

Lie on your back, one pillow under your head, knees bent up, feet on the bed. Pull your tummy in, tighten your pelvic floor, tilt your bottom upwards slightly and try to press the middle of your back flat against the mattress. Hold briefly, then relax. Do not hold your breath and do not press down on your feet. Repeat five times, at least three times daily. Try this pelvic tilting movement in a sitting position as well as while standing and walking, to correct your posture. This exercise should ease backache and help to reduce flatulence (wind) (Figure 15).

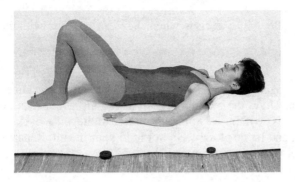

Figure 15   *Pelvic tilting.*

As an additional exercise, pull your tummy in and hold for a few seconds, then let go slowly. Remember to keep breathing normally. Do this exercise frequently in all positions, including walking.

Knee Rolling

Lie on your back with your knees bent up, feet on the bed, one pillow under your head. Pull your tummy in. With knees together, slowly roll your knees first to one side and then to the other, a few inches to each side (Figure 16). This exercise, done gently and rhythmically in a 'tic-toc' movement, may also relieve flatulence.

Figure 16
Knee rolling.

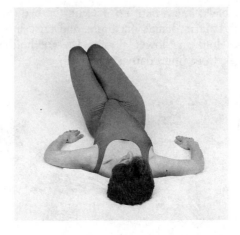

21

ADDITIONAL EXERCISES AFTER YOUR STITCHES ARE OUT, OR ONE WEEK AFTER VAGINAL REPAIR OR COLPOSUSPENSION

(Only do the following exercises when they can be done without causing pain or discomfort.)

Hip Hitching

Lying on your back, head on pillow, one leg straight, one knee bent up, pull tummy in. Draw the straight leg up at the hip to make it shorter by about 2–3 inches, without bending the knee, sliding the back of the leg along the bed, and let go slowly. Do not hold your breath. Repeat six times each side, three times daily (Figure 17).

Figure 17
Hip hitching.

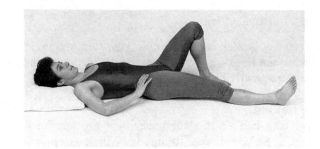

Head Raising

Lying on your back, knees bent up, feet on the bed, head on pillow, pull tummy in, tuck chin in, hands on thighs and raise head off the pillow to look at knees. Hold and lower slowly. Do not hold your breath. Rest. Repeat six times, three times daily (Figure 18).

Figure 18
Head raising.

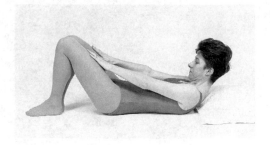

Head Raising with Hand to Opposite Knee

Lying on your back, pillow under head, knees bent up, feet on the bed, arms straight and away from side. Pull tummy in, raise head, tuck chin in, lift straight arm and reach over to touch opposite thigh or knee, and return to starting position. Do not hold your breath. Rest. Repeat on opposite side. Do this exercise three times on each side, increasing gradually to six times on each side (Figure 19).

Figure 19
Head raising with hand to opposite knee.

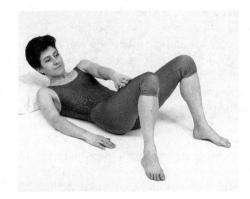

Knee Rolling (continued)

Position as above. With tummy pulled in, roll knees to one side as far as is comfortable, return to central position and repeat to opposite side. Do not hold your breath. Repeat six times, three times daily.

AFTER LEAVING HOSPITAL

The majority of patients are well enough to leave hospital a few days after their operation. This varies according to your individual rate of recovery, the advice of your doctor and the method and extent of the surgery performed. As already mentioned, although externally the scar will heal quickly, usually within a week, the internal healing process takes considerably longer.

The recovery time is very important. Resting and following the advice carefully will ensure that the tissues heal correctly – and *remember* that the success of your operation depends on this.

Rest and Exercise

When you go home you will need at least a week's extended 'hospital' care. That means resting, getting up when you want to, relaxing and – of course – continuing with the exercises.

Try to avoid standing still for more than a few minutes at a time. If you keep your legs moving it will help your circulation.

You may find you tire easily. Do not worry about this. The return to normal life following any major operation takes time and is a gradual process. In general, do what you feel you sensibly can.

The pelvic floor exercise is important for women of all ages. Do it just as regularly after leaving hospital. You would be wise to continue doing it for the rest of your life, as it is one of the best ways in which a woman can maintain urinary control. If you think you will forget, associate the pelvic floor exercise with an everyday activity such as turning on a tap or a switch and do it then. Also, try to remember to do it when you cough or sneeze.

Personal Cleanliness

This continues to be important once you have left hospital. A daily bath is recommended. If only a shower is available, you should pay special attention to cleaning the genital area, but douching is *not* advisable.

Diet

A well-balanced nutritious diet containing a high fibre content is essential to avoid constipation. Eat plenty of fresh fruit, salads, green vegetables and wholemeal bread. Try to make sure you get enough food that contains protein, such as meat, eggs and fish, or pulses (peas, beans, lentils) if you are a vegetarian. Avoid fried and stodgy foods, cakes, pastries, sweets and chocolate. Drink plenty of fluids – at least one litre a day.

Constipation

This is frequently a problem following pelvic surgery, due to having a diet low in roughage and also a lack of exercise. As already mentioned, straining to pass a motion can be harmful and should be avoided. If a laxative is required, mild natural remedies such as lactulose or Senokot are recommended.

Weight Control

There is no reason why you should gain weight following a hysterectomy. If you follow the advice given for diet, and take gradually increased regular exercise, you should stay at your normal weight.

Walking

Walking is the perfect exercise. When you go home you should aim for a 10-minute walk daily, gradually increasing to a 30-45 minute walk by four weeks, or two short walks if you prefer. But remember – only walk the distance that you can achieve comfortably.

Stairs

It is quite safe to go up and down stairs from about the fourth day after your operation (Figure 20).

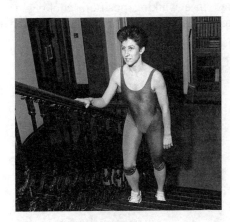

Figure 20 *Going up stairs: back straight, weight forward, hold handrail.*

Fatigue and Vulnerability

Many people find that they tire easily after surgery – it is important to recognise that this is normal.

Don't push yourself too hard too soon! Don't feel anxious if you find this tiredness continues for some weeks. Don't persist with any activity that you cannot achieve easily. Only you know how much you can do, and everyone is individual. You will gain strength gradually, so if you find the guidelines for activity and exercise suggested in the booklet are difficult to achieve, give yourself an extra day or two and try again. Remember, always extend activities slowly and at the pace your body dictates.

Women may also feel emotionally vulnerable for a while – it is reassuring to know that this is a common experience. Your morale will improve as your recovery progresses. The help and understanding of family and friends, if you are fortunate enough to have this support, can be invaluable at this time.

The convalescent period is a very important time and your body must be given time to heal. You must progress at your own rate. Don't feel a failure because you know of others who have recovered more quickly.

Housework

Have a rest for the first few days you are at home. However, you can make a cup of tea, help with washing up, dusting and easy household jobs, etc. Reduce your standing. Sit on a stool or chair whenever possible.

About three weeks after your operation you can gradually start to do more household jobs, such as using a light vacuum cleaner with your feet apart in a walking position, cooking, ironing etc. (Figure 21), with the exception of work involving heavy lifting or prolonged standing.

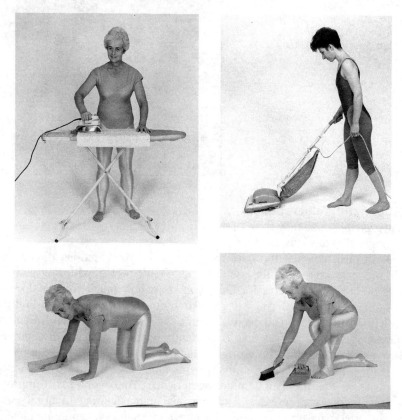

Figure 21   *Housework: (a) Ironing – note correct height of ironing board; (b) Vacuuming – feet apart in a walking position; (c) Cleaning the floor – use same position for weeding; (d) Using dustpan and brush.*

26

Lifting

For the first four weeks reduce lifting wherever possible to allow the tissues to heal correctly and avoid future damage. As a guide, do not lift more than a full 3-pint kettle of water or its equivalent, i.e. 3–4 kg or 6–8 lbs. Heavy lifting or moving furniture should not be attempted until *at least* 8–10 weeks after surgery. Following colposuspension, heavy lifting must never be attempted again.

Remember: When you do lift, do it correctly. With your feet placed firmly apart in the walking position, bend your knees, back straight, pull in tummy and tighten pelvic floor muscles, hold the object to be lifted or carried close to you, and lift by straightening your knees (Figure 22).

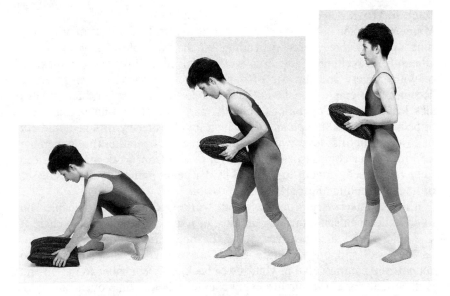

Figure 22   *How to lift correctly: (a) Bend knees, back straight, pull tummy in, tighten pelvic floor muscles, hold object to be lifted close to you; (b) Lift by straightening your knees; (c) Back straight, holding object close to you.*

Driving

To get into a car comfortably, stand with the back of your legs close to the car seat, bend forwards from the hips, bend your knees and sit backwards into the car seat using your hand on the car door frame to steady yourself. Pull in your tummy muscles and lift first one leg and then the other slowly into the car. Remember – do not twist your back. Get out of the car in the same way, but always stand up straight before walking away.

It is usually safe to drive a car at about three weeks following surgery, although after any operation this will depend on your confidence and concentration, and also on your ability to do an emergency stop. But – check first that your car insurance policy does not have an exclusion relating to major surgery.

Concentration

Many women find their ability to concentrate is affected following surgery for a variable length of time.

Back to Work

Your own doctor will advise you when to return to work. It may be any time up to twelve weeks, depending on the type of work you do, the amount of travelling to and from work involved, and of course the extent of your surgery and the rate of your recovery. However, it is generally accepted that employers should be prepared to allow up to three months sick leave for these operations. Initially, part-time or flexi-hours may have to be negotiated, although any job which involves heavy lifting should *not* be resumed until at least twelve weeks after your operation (but remember *no* lifting after colposuspension). Travel to and from work may also need to be reassessed – a door-to-door lift by car being preferable to the stresses of travel by public transport, if at all possible.

It may be necessary to reassess your working conditions, to enable you to sit rather than stand for long periods, or request a more suitable chair. If you have a job which involves sitting for long periods, do make sure your back is well supported (Figure 23). If necessary, use a small pillow to support the natural curve in your lower back, and remember to get up and walk around for a few minutes every couple of hours. Employers and work colleagues, particularly males, may not always appreciate the implications of your recent surgery and may need educating! You may also need to be assertive to ensure your future health and full recovery – if necessary supported by a letter from your doctor. Try to discuss your operation and its implications with your manager/boss before your operation.

Sport and Activity Hobbies

The rate of recovery from surgery varies for everyone. As a guide, it should be safe to start about 8–10 weeks after the operation (not before 10 weeks

Figure 23   *Sitting at a desk: back supported, feet flat on floor.*

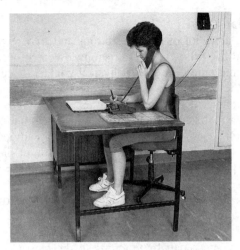

following colposuspension), or earlier for regular exercisers, following the approval of the doctor at your post-operative check. Exercise classes at a beginner's standard, if these are available at a local leisure centre, or a specially tailored training programme by a qualified instructor, would be a good way to begin a gradual return to fitness. It is important to follow the pace your body dictates and not to push yourself beyond your ability to cope comfortably. A gentle return is essential.

Only begin with those activities that can be stopped at any point when you feel tired. A gradual build-up to competitive games is advisable.

Warning. **Never try to do the following while lying on your back:** (i) lifting both legs together while straight; and (ii) 'sit-ups' with legs straight.

Digging or any heavy garden work which involves lifting must not be attempted until at least twelve weeks following surgery (and is not advisable at all after colposuspension). However, it is possible to do easier garden jobs at an earlier stage – for example, from about three to six weeks, hand weeding and planting out small plants kneeling on all fours, or light hoeing with your feet apart in a walking stance, avoiding any twisting movements. Do not push yourself.

Gentle swimming for pleasure can usually be started after two to three weeks, providing any discharge has stopped. At first choose a quiet time when there are few people in the pool.

If there are any doubts or special circumstances, ask your doctor for advice.

Sexual Activity

There are a lot of misconceptions and 'old wives' tales' about a woman's sexual life following hysterectomy. Women need love and affection at this time and enjoy the close physical contact of cuddling and touching. They and their partners often request specific advice about resuming sexual intercourse. If the opportunity exists, it may be helpful for you and your partner to discuss the operation with a health professional beforehand.

In order to understand exactly what advice we give and why, it is important first of all to understand a little of the female anatomy and how the reproductive organs are affected during the operation (see Figures 1, 2 3 and 4).

The vagina is just a passage into which protrudes the cervix (entrance to the womb). As already described, during hysterectomy the womb and usually the cervix as well are removed. This obviously involves some surgery and repair by stitching to the far end of the vagina. Initially, this shortens the passage very slightly, but as the vagina is lined with folds of stretchy skin, this should create no problem when sexual intercourse is resumed. This depends very much on the extent of the vaginal surgery, the rate of healing and the couple's own preference.

Many women prefer to wait until after the post-operative check (usually about six weeks) to be sure the area is completely healed. This is because sexual arousal (not only intercourse) tends to have a stretching effect on the vagina which could interfere with the healing process. Once this area is completely healed, sexual activity may be resumed.

Because the size and angle of the vagina may have been altered slightly, it may be wise to try out different positions for intercourse to find how you are most comfortable.

Obviously, your husband or sexual partner should be gentle at first. It may also help considerably to use a proprietary lubricant such as K-Y Jelly (obtainable from any chemist). This is because the vagina may not produce enough natural lubrication while you are tense or apprehensive about resuming sexual activity.

Most women find it reassuring to know that their own sexual response should be very little changed by the operation, since the external reproductive organs are unaltered. If a climax is normally experienced, this will still be possible.

SMEAR TESTS

Women who have undergone a hysterectomy frequently enquire about continuing with 'smear tests'. Where the womb, including the cervix, has been removed, *cervical* smears are no longer possible. Where a 'sub-total' hysterectomy has been performed, the cervix remains and smears should continue to be taken. If the womb has been removed because of abnormal cervical smears or cancer, the consultant may wish to continue to observe and take occasional smears from the 'vaginal vault' – the deepest part of the vagina.

THE MENOPAUSE (Climacteric or Change of Life)

Many women undergoing hysterectomy and/or vaginal repair ask questions about the menopause, and they may also require information regarding hormone replacement therapy.

The word 'menopause' really means 'last period', but we use it to describe the changes which happen to a woman's body around this time of life. The menopause is a normal body function that usually occurs at about the age of fifty, but which can happen both earlier and later than this. There is often a familial tendency – mother and daughter frequently following a similar menopausal pattern.

Menopausal symptoms are caused by a decrease in the hormone levels produced by the ovaries as they cease to function. These symptoms can also result from the surgical removal of both ovaries which sometimes accompanies hysterectomy (Figures 1 and 2). The fall in production of these hormones – oestrogen and progesterone – can affect the body in the following areas:

Firstly, the muscles and nerves which control the blood vessels – this may produce the hot flushes, night sweats, palpitations and headaches which some menopausal women experience to a varying degree.

For those women who have *not* undergone hysterectomy, periods become irregular and eventually cease altogether. Many women welcome the end to a monthly inconvenience, enjoying the freedom from discomfort, bleeding and the expense of purchasing sanitary protection. Vaginal dryness may be experienced, so that sexual intercourse without additional lubrication (such as K-Y Jelly, already mentioned) becomes uncomfortable – and consequently the desire to make love may lessen.

The skin, hair and bones can also be influenced by these hormonal changes – the skin becoming dryer, hair less greasy, thinning and changing in texture. Bones may gradually lose their density, become more brittle and so break more easily. The areas most vulnerable are the wrist and the weight-carrying bones of the leg. This condition is called osteoporosis and is greatly helped by the use of HRT (see next section), although a calcium-rich diet and regular exercise are also thought to be of great value.

The degree to which each individual woman is affected by these changes, and the time taken in passing through the menopause, varies enormously, with the majority of women experiencing very little discomfort. It is helpful at this time to choose cotton rather than synthetic materials – particularly underwear, nightclothes and bed linen. Light layers of clothing which are easily removed and replaced are more comfortable than thick heavy garments. Tepid rather than hot showers and baths are preferable. Indeed it may temporarily be best to avoid any situations which are hot, airless or crowded.

It is also advisable to avoid alcohol, as well as hot and spicy foods (such as curry, chilli con carne, etc.) and to reduce caffeine intake, i.e. tea and coffee.

Additional 'self-help' measures may help to lessen menopausal symptoms. A sensible life style including regular exercise has already been mentioned, and practising relaxation may also be beneficial. Find time to follow your own interests. A well-balanced nutritious diet including particularly the foods rich in calcium, i.e. milk, cheese etc., is thought to be helpful at this time.

Some women, however, find the menopause a very difficult and lengthy process, with both physical and psychological problems to overcome. Coping with hot flushes, sweats and sexual discomfort may give rise to psychological symptoms such as depression, sleeplessness, loss of energy or confidence, and irritability. Where menopausal symptoms are causing severe discomfort, or affecting family relationships or work ability, the situation may be improved by sympathetic professional counselling (which may be obtained at local Well Women clinics), understanding family support, and possibly hormone replacement therapy.

HORMONE REPLACEMENT THERAPY (HRT)

If the ovaries are *both* removed, the doctor may advise replacing artificially the hormones that the ovaries normally produce. HRT may also be prescribed to help relieve symptoms experienced when undergoing a natural menopause and help to prevent osteoporosis and heart disease.

Hormone Replacement Therapy

HRT is most commonly given in the form of tablets taken daily or as instructed. The tablets may be supplied in a 'calendar' pack similar to the contraceptive pill – older women may need reassurance about any risks involved in taking HRT, especially if they were advised to discontinue the contraceptive pill in their mid-30s. HRT is now very sophisticated and involves much smaller doses than in the contraceptive pill, although it contains the same female hormones.

However, your doctor may prefer to give HRT in the form of a 'slow release' implant placed under the skin (usually of the abdominal wall or buttock) and renewed approximately every six months, or as required. This is a very simple painless procedure where the doctor slips the implant through a small 'nick' in the skin, under local anaesthetic. The first implant is often inserted when the hysterectomy is actually performed, especially if it is carried out before the menopause.

HRT is also available in the form of 'patches' which enable the hormone to be absorbed through the skin. These are small, round hormone-impregnated adhesive discs, one of which is applied to the skin below the waist – usually the outer thigh or buttock – and changed twice a week. They are not disturbed by baths or showers and are a convenient form of HRT, although some women experience a local skin reaction and irritation caused by the patch adhesive.

Local applications in the form of skin gels or vaginal creams may also be prescribed, but these should not be used immediately prior to or as a lubricant for intercourse, as these female hormones may be absorbed by the male partner.

Women who have not had a hysterectomy may continue to have a monthly bleed while taking HRT (depending on the medication prescribed), but are not at risk of pregnancy once the ovaries are no longer functioning. The length of time for which HRT will be prescribed depends upon the needs of each individual. Your doctor should explain this more fully.

Every woman for whom HRT is prescribed, whether by mouth, local application or implant, should continue to be monitored by medical super-vision. This will involve periodic blood pressure checks and smear tests for women who still have their cervix. Being 'breast aware' is also important.

IN CONCLUSION

A hysterectomy, vaginal repair or colposuspension should remove the cause of some miserable, painful, uncomfortable and debilitating symptoms. By giving full and accurate information on the surgery and its effect, and thus alleviating much of the anxiety associated with the operation, we hope this booklet will enable you to look forward to a new lease of life.

However, every woman is individual and it is important that you should ask for a full explanation of the diagnosis or suggested surgery in your own particular case. Do not be afraid to ask questions of your consultant, the hospital medical, nursing or physiotherapy staff, or your own GP or practice nurse. By fully understanding your own problem, unnecessary anxiety will be prevented and you will make a speedier and more confident recovery.

USEFUL ADDRESSES

Amarant Centre (advice on hormone replacement therapy), 80 Lambeth Road, London SE1 7PW. Tel. 0171–401 3855

Association of Chartered Physiotherapists in Women's Health, c/o The Chartered Society of Physiotherapy, 14 Bedford Row, London WC1R 4ED. Tel. 0171–306 6666.

BACUP (advice and counselling for cancer patients and their families), 3 Bath Place, Rivington Street, London EC2A 3JR. Tel. (free) 0800–181199

British Association for Counselling, 1 Regent Place, Rugby CV21 2PJ. Tel. 01788–578328

Continence Foundation, 2 Doughty Street, London WC1N 2PH. Tel. 0171–404 6875.

Endometriosis Society, 35 Belgrave Square, London SW1X 8QB. Tel. 0171–235 4137

Family Planning Association, 2–12 Pentonville Road, London N1 9FP. Tel. 0171–837 5432

Hysterectomy Support Network, 3 Lynne Close, Green Street Green, Orpington, Kent BR6 6BS.

National Osteoporosis Society, P.O. Box 10, Radstock, Bath BA3 3YB. Tel. 01761–471771.

Additional Reading

Women's Health, 52 Featherstone Street, London EC1Y 8RT.
Tel. 0171–251 6580
Women's Health Concern (WHC). Send SAE with your enquiry to WHC
at: 83 Earl's Court Road, London W8 6EF.
Women's Nationwide Cancer Control Campaign, Suna House,
128–130 Curtain Road, London EC2A 3AR.
Tel. 0171–729 4688; helpline 0171–729 2229.

ADDITIONAL READING

Endometriosis, Suzie Hayman, Thorsons.
Everywoman: a Gynaecological Guide for Life, Derek Llewellyn-Jones,
Penguin.
Fibroids, Felicity Smart and Stuart Campbell, Thorsons.
Having a Cervical Smear, Sally Haslett, Beaconsfield.
Having Gynaecological Surgery, Sally Haslett and Molly Jennings,
Beaconsfield.
Hormone Replacement Therapy: Making Your Own Decision, Patsy
Westcott, Thorsons.
HRT and the Menopause, National Osteoporosis Society.
Hysterectomy, Susie Hayman, Sheldon Press.
*Hysterectomy: A Reassuring Guide to Surgery, Recovery and Your
Choices*, Jane Butterworth, Thorsons.
Hysterectomy: New Options and Advances, Lorraine Dennerstein, Carl
Wood and Ann Westmore, Oxford University Press.
Let's Get Moving: Overcoming Constipation, Pauline Chiarelli, Health
Books.
Menopause, The, Family Planning Association.
Woman's Guide to Surgery, The, Tim Coltart and Felicity Smart,
Thorsons.
Women's Waterworks: Curing Incontinence, Pauline Chiarelli, Health
Books.

Books marked with an asterisk are available by mail order from Family
Planning Association Book Sales, 2–12 Pentonville Road, London, N1
9FP. Tel. 0171–923 5215; Fax 0171–837 3026.

Acknowledgements

We would like to acknowledge with many thanks our indebtedness to the following for their help and support:

The medical, nursing and senior physiotherapy staff at St Thomas' Hospital, London, for their advice and cooperation in the original development of this booklet.

The following persons and members of the relevant professional groups, all of whom made time to read a late draft of this Fourth Edition and give us their detailed comments, which we were very pleased to be able to take into account when preparing the final version for press: Professor Linda Cardozo, Professor Stuart Stanton, Ms Kathy Bryson, Ms Bridget Gill, Ms Angela Reid and Ms Vicky Smiley, Ms Vicki Allanach and the members of the Executive Committee of the Gynaecological Forum of the Royal College of Nursing, and Ms Jill Mantle and her colleagues on the Education Sub-Committee of the Association of Chartered Physiotherapists in Women's Health.

S.H., M.J.